The Ten Best Essential Oils

Desk Reference Guide

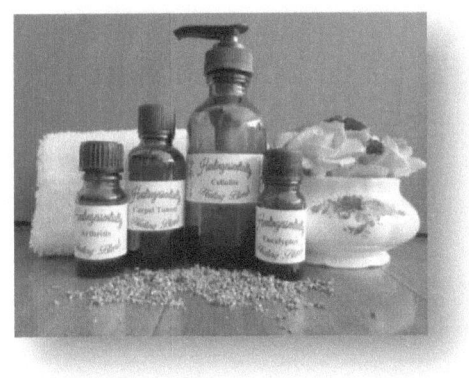

Kate Richardson

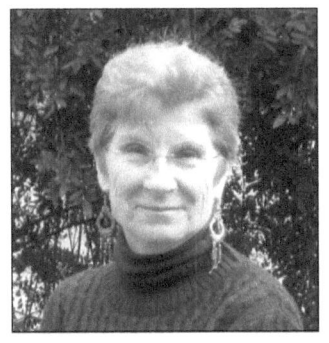

The Author is a Natural Therapist with a practice in Tasmania, Australia.

Her range of modalities include Huna Massage, Reflexology, Aromatherapy Massage, Ear Candling, Herbal Bodywraps and Tarot Card Readings. She is a Registered Trainer and qualified practitioner of these healing arts.

An awareness of Essential Oils for the Aromatherapy Massage quickly became an extensive interest as the scope of the properties and versatility of using essential oils in healing became evident.

Amazement at the ability of the essential oils on their own or in a synergistic blend to promote the wellbeing of the body and emotional peace of the soul convinced the Author that these natural products are the future (as they were for the past) of the health industry.

The intention of this book is to provide a comprehensive Reference Guide which lists the best, most useful and readily available essential oils, the ways to use them and which carrier oils will be the best to combine with the appropriate oils to aid in healing the body, easing the mind, protecting the home and reducing the chemical footprint on the planet.

Please refer to the website
www.healingessentially.com
for more information and recipes

Contents

Introduction

There are around 300 essential oils which could be used to heal, cleanse or protect our health and homes. But are they all vital for home use?

No, not really…

If you are interested in having a basic kit or first aid box of essential oils for your family then there really are only about 10 essential oils that would be necessary. These 10 essential oils are so versatile, adaptable and have so many wonderful qualities – which can be used on their own or in conjunction with each other – that most household and family needs will be more than adequately covered.

You will probably have heard of all of these 10 best essential oils before – they are so popular because they are so versatile. And for those of us in Australia **Eucalyptus** is very familiar – most of us have grown up with it in the house with our mums reaching for it when the usual seasonal coughs and colds hit the kids.

Although the therapeutic value of most essential oils ceases after about two years the disinfectant ability of Eucalyptus oil just gets better, so once it is past the two years use it in your kitchen cleaning bottle instead of your healing blends to disinfect the kitchen shelves and benches.

Lavender runs a close second with its strong antiseptic qualities. A spray bottle of lavender in the house is fantastic for refreshing the air as well as eliminating odours and scaring off the bugs.

Peppermint essential oil we all know from the confectionary aisle of any supermarket but that is purely a chemical imitation of the real thing and pales into insignificance beside the pure essential oil.

All of the essential oils listed here are easily available from reputable suppliers.

Remember to always store your essential oils away from heat and light, in a blue or amber bottle with a tight seal to avoid evaporation.

Don't store your bottles for a long time with a dripolator in the lid as this rubber or plastic could perish and contaminate your oils.

Very importantly, always store your essential oils out of the children's reach.

Lastly, if you want to make your own essential oil blends for general use or massage just remember that the ratio of essential oils to each other in any blend is the key to the success of that particular blend. Just adding a drop of this and a dash of that and giving the whole thing a shake is not necessarily going to have the desired effect.

Note: Do not take essential oils internally without the advice of a qualified Aromatherapist.

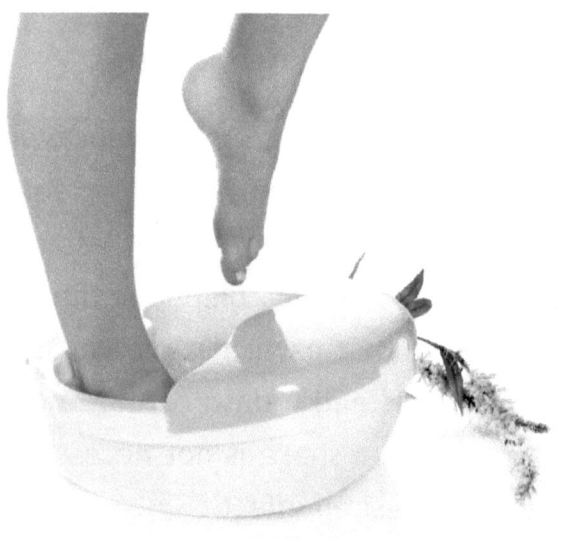

Chapter 1

Methods to Use Essential Oils

Pure essential oils are strong chemicals and should not be applied directly to the skin. They can cause skin irritations, burning sensation or a tingling feeling. There are some exceptions like **Lavender** which can be applied directly to burns, scalds, cuts, insect bites or cramps. **Tea Tree** can also be applied directly to cure Athlete's Foot, warts and nail infections.

Other essential oils need to be diluted in a carrier oil. The normal maximum dilution rate for adults is 30 drops to 30 millilitres of carrier oil.

It is not recommended to use essential oils during pregnancy unless under a qualified Aromatherapist's care.

To use with children it is recommended to use at least half the ratio of an adult, and not to use on small babies at all.

➢ _Baths_:

You can't go past a soak in the tub! If essential oils are added to the water then you have the therapeutic benefit of whichever oils you have chosen – they can be combined for relaxation or stimulation.

You can use the essential oils neat, that is, a few drops of the oils directly into the hot water or you can add the oils via a carrier oil – but in this case the oil may cling to your skin a little.

Either way it will be of immense benefit and enjoyment to inhale the aroma whilst relaxing and feeling the oils being absorbed into your skin.

If neat use about 3 - 4 drops, if diluted in carrier oil pour about a teaspoon into the water. Soak for as long as you want, but at least 15 minutes.

➢ _Footbaths_:

Soak your tired feet in a footbath with hot water and the essential oil of choice. Relax and allow the oils to penetrate the soles of your feet for maximum benefit.

If you have particularly sore or aching feet place some smooth or round small stones in the base of the footbath and fill it to cover your ankles and then, after adding the essential oils, roll your feet over the stones to ease those tight muscles.

Then use a pumice stone and gently but firmly rub this over the softened skin to remove the dead cells. Use **Peppermint** for refreshing your feet or **Geranium** for circulation.

Oils: 2-6 drops.

➢ *Hand baths*:

To ease sore or painful joints place some **Chamomile** in hot water and soak your hands for as long as it is comfortable.

For dry hands you can use **Geranium**, for work worn hands use **Lemon** and to cleanse hands use **Lavender** or **Eucalyptus**.

Oils: 2-4 drops.

➢ *Sitz bath*:

Use either a sitz bath or fill a bathtub to only allow the lower half of the body to be covered. Add the essential oils of choice and mix thoroughly.

It will depend on the condition to be treated as to what essential oils are used.   Possible essential oils here could be **Tea Tree** for Cystitis and **Geranium** for Haemorrhoids.

Oils: 2-3 drops.

➢ *Compresses*:

Hot Compress: Use a bowl of hot water and the essential oils to treat muscular aches, arthritic conditions, menstrual pain, cystitis, frozen shoulder. Soak a cloth in this water and apply to the affected area.

Cold Compress: Use a bowl of cold water with ice and the essential oils to help reduce swelling in conditions like bruises, boils, headaches, fever.

➢ *Diffusers*:

These are purpose built tools which use heat (candle flame, electricity, whatever) to disperse the essential oil into the atmosphere. Another name for diffusers is Burners.

The ideal uses for this method are meditation, a memory aid or stress, where you are able to sit quietly in a room away from distractions.

Remember to clean off the residue from the previous use as the essential oils may cross contaminate each other and produce the wrong result for your purpose.

Oils: 1-6 drops.

> ## _Gargling:_

For the treatment of mouth ulcers, sore throat or bad breath add essential oil to a glass of warm water and gargle.

Oils: 2 drops. Repeat as necessary.

> ## _Inhalation via Vapour:_

Pour boiling hot water into a large bowl, add the essential oils of choice, like **Eucalyptus**, cover your head with a towel and inhale the vapour.

The idea behind this method is to allow the steam to penetrate deeper areas of the head and throat so it is perfect for colds, flu, sinusitis and sore throat.

Keep doing it until you feel the congestion is easing, may take 10 – 15 minutes. Repeat as necessary.

Oils: 1-3 drops.

➤ *Inhalation via Tissue*:

Place the drop of essential oil on a tissue and inhale. This method is excellent for insomnia as the tissue is placed on the pillow and you can breathe in the oil as you drift off to sleep. Try a couple of drops of **Lavender**.

Also excellent for colds and flu as you can hold the tissue up against your nose and breathe deeply of the essential oil, particularly good for stuffy noses. Use **Eucalyptus** here.

Oils: 1-2 drops. Repeat as necessary.

> ➤ *Jacuzzi*:

Essential oils are just great in a Jacuzzi but be mindful of spreading diseases or germs through the water if you are sharing the Jacuzzi so the best oils to use would be the anti-fungal and anti-viral essential oils of **Eucalyptus**, **Lavender** and **Thyme**.

Oils: 3 drops per person.

> ➤ *Massage*:

One of the best and most popular ways to gain the maximum benefit from essential oils is via a massage; a full body massage especially.

There are so many possibilities for massage oils or blends that it is really up to you what you like to have or what you feel the need for in a massage.

The combination of touch and healing with the therapeutic benefits of the essential oils make this modality a firm favourite with everyone.

> ## *Room Sprays*:

Use a spray bottle which hasn't been used for anything else and always keep it for the essential oil room spray of your choice.

Fill the spray bottle with water, add a few drops of the essential oil or oils, shake gently and spray the room. It is especially useful in a sickroom to freshen up the room or eliminate germs.

It is also good for bathrooms to eliminate odours. But it is great just for any room in the house – use **Lavender** for a disinfectant and room freshener.

Oils: 4 drops per 300ml of water.

> *Sauna*:

Mix the essential oils of choice and sprinkle on the hot stones. The best oils for saunas are those which are anti-toxins like **Eucalyptus** and **Tea Tree** – these essential oils will help remove the toxins via sweating.

Oils: 2-4 drops

> *Shower*:

After showering place the essential oils of choice on a face cloth and rub it gently over the whole body while the water is still running. Breathe in deeply. Bliss! Any oils here would be fine – choose for aroma.

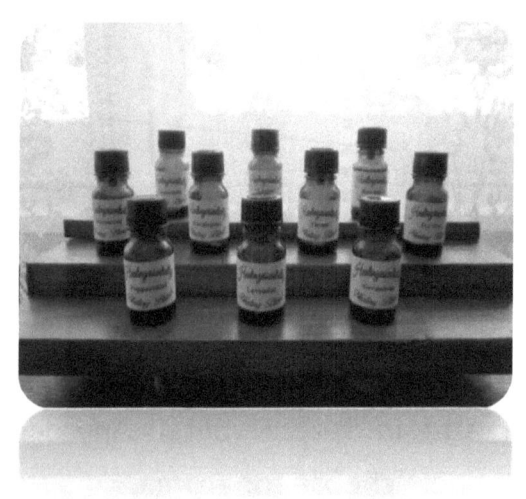

Chapter 2

The 10 Best Essential Oils

Chamomile (matricaria recutita)

Chamomile has two main types: German and Roman. They are structurally different in their compounds but the medicinal properties are very similar. Although Chamomile has many uses and benefits such as being anti-bacterial, an antiseptic and a disinfectant the prime attribute of Chamomile is as an anti-inflammatory. This covers both internal conditions such as rheumatism/arthritis and also external like burns, psoriasis, eczema, sprains.

Chamomile is extremely effective in calming and soothing the mind so use it for nervous tension, depression, insomnia, headaches, releasing emotional blockages, controlling anger.

For getting off tranquillisers it's the perfect solution!

Its soothing qualities can be used externally as well for acne, burns, cuts and any dry and itchy skin conditions.

The methods of use are up to you, depending on what you need it for. For skin conditions use it as a topical application; for soothing the mind it can be used in the bath or maybe in a burner; if you have a sprain then a compress is the way to go.

Source:

Flowers via Distillation

Properties:

- ➤ Analgesic
- ➤ Antibacterial
- ➤ Antispasmodic
- ➤ Anti-inflammatory
- ➤ Sedative

<u>Uses</u>:

- ➢ Abscesses & Toothache
- ➢ Acne
- ➢ Arthritis
- ➢ Asthma
- ➢ Anxiety
- ➢ Boils
- ➢ Burns & Blisters
- ➢ Bursitis
- ➢ Cold Sores
- ➢ Dermatitis
- ➢ Eczema
- ➢ HayFever
- ➢ Headache
- ➢ Infections
- ➢ Nervousness
- ➢ Muscle Cramps

<u>Caution</u>

Avoid if you are allergic to the ragweed family

Eucalyptus (Eucalyptus Globulus)

There are over 700 varieties of Eucalyptus, however not all are used for aromatherapy. The scent comes from the core compound, eucalyptol, which is common in all varieties.

Eucalyptus has been used for thousands of years by the Australian Aboriginals for its medicinal properties. It has been a household favourite in Australia for many years. Eucalyptus is particularly effective as a decongestant so use it specifically for all respiratory ailments like the cold and flu viruses.

It has wonderful fever reducing qualities and strong anti-inflammatory and antibiotic attributes so is an invaluable aid in the sickroom. Use it as a room spray to eliminate bacteria and microbes.

It is useful in a topical application for cuts, blisters, cold sores, abscesses, stings/bites.

As a massage preparation it is used extensively for many health conditions including but not limited to: muscular aches and pains, arthritis, poor circulation, nervous tension, headaches.

As a memory boost use it in a burner or bath, as a mood enhancer it is fantastic to lighten and revitalise our sense of wellbeing.

Source:

Leaves via distillation

Properties:

- ➢ Antibacterial
- ➢ Antiseptic
- ➢ Antispasmodic
- ➢ Antiviral
- ➢ Antibiotic
- ➢ Analgesic
- ➢ Decongestant
- ➢ Diuretic
- ➢ Deodorant
- ➢ Expectorant

<u>Uses</u>:

- Acne
- Arthritis
- Asthma
- Boils
- Bronchitis & Colds
- Bruises
- Burns & Blister
- Cooling
- Cystitis
- Candida
- Headaches
- Insect Repellent
- Muscular Aches
- Neuralgia
- Sunburn
- Stings & Insect Bites
- Throat Infections

Geranium (Pelargonium Graveolens)

Geranium is considered a general all-rounder essential oil with multiples applications and a delightful aroma.

Because of its cell regenerating and hormone balancing abilities Geranium is excellent for all skin types: moisturising dry skin, maintaining the balance of normal skin and adjusting oily skin. These attributes will be helpful in skin conditions as well eg acne, wrinkles, eczema. Used in skin care products it can give a lovely glow to the skin, refreshing in a cologne or face splash and revitalising for tired skin.

One of Geranium's key properties is its ability to balance hormones so it can be very effective for all those difficult times for ladies: teenage years, heavy periods, premenstrual syndrome and menopausal symptoms.

Geranium is an excellent aid in reducing chilblains, it is an excellent component in the treatment of endometriosis, a tonic for the liver, an aid in stimulating blood circulation, improves the flow of lymph and is a good treatment for herpes, shingles, burns, haemorrhoids. You can use it as an insect repellent and with its anti-fungal properties use it as a topical application for ringworm and other viral or fungal infections of the skin.

Geranium's scent is wonderful for those times when we are a little sad or depressed, needing a lift. Use it in a burner or bath to settle the mind, ease the spirit, nurture your soul.

Source:

Leaves, flowers, stalks via distillation

Properties:

- ➤ Antibacterial
- ➤ Antidepressant
- ➤ Antiseptic
- ➤ Astringent
- ➤ Sedative

<u>Uses</u>:

- ➢ Acne
- ➢ Bruises
- ➢ Burns & Cuts
- ➢ Calming
- ➢ Chilblains
- ➢ Herpes
- ➢ Insect Repellent
- ➢ Facial Splashes
- ➢ Fungal Infections
- ➢ Oedema
- ➢ Liver Tonic
- ➢ Poor Circulation
- ➢ Sedative
- ➢ Stretch Marks
- ➢ Throat Infections

Lavender (Lavandula Angustifolia)

A perennial favourite and one of the best known, both for its lovely scent, and its distinctive colour.

One of the main uses for Lavender is for burns or scalds as it seems to speed healing and reduces scarring by stimulating the cells to regenerate more quickly. Wonderful stuff, particularly for inquisitive children! A must for every parent to have a bottle of Lavender handy.

Not only burns and scalds but bites, stings, grazes and other little nasties that happen in a day to small children or big adults –all will be helped by using Lavender.

A spin off from applying to a burn is the calming effect of the Lavender to the emotional shock of the injury.

Lavender's antibacterial and antiseptic qualities make it helpful in inflammatory conditions of the skin like acne and its decongestant properties make it effective for all coughs, colds or flu symptoms.

One of the most popular uses for Lavender is for improving sleep. Combine it with Valerian and you won't need sleeping pills anymore!

Source:

Flowers via distillation

Properties:

- ➢ Analgesic
- ➢ Antibacterial
- ➢ Antibiotic
- ➢ Anti-depressant
- ➢ Antispasmodic
- ➢ Antiseptic
- ➢ Anti-inflammatory
- ➢ Decongestant

Uses:

- ➢ Acne
- ➢ Asthma
- ➢ Bites & Stings
- ➢ Burns & Scalds
- ➢ Cell Stimulant
- ➢ Colds & Coughs
- ➢ Eczema
- ➢ Exhaustion
- ➢ Grazes
- ➢ Insect Repellent
- ➢ Insomnia
- ➢ Labour & Period Pain
- ➢ Muscle Aches
- ➢ Sciatica
- ➢ Scars
- ➢ Sinusitis
- ➢ Stress

Caution:

Don't use if you have very Low Blood Pressure

Lemon (Citrus Limonum)

Lemon is wonderful in essential oil blends as a synergistic agent which is one of the reasons it is used so frequently in blends. However, it does have a multitude of qualities of its own. Everyone has probably heard about its ability to prevent scurvy!

It is also an excellent tonic for the lymphatic system by helping to stimulate the growth of lymphocytes which support your body's immune system. By improving the lymphatic circulation Lemon will help you slim, help fight respiratory ailments like flu or a cold, viral infections like herpes, and with its strong antiseptic qualities it's very useful in healing cuts and scrapes.

Lemon is also an aid in reducing high blood pressure while its detoxifying abilities help shift cellulite, ease painful joints, boost blood circulation and stimulate the digestive system.

Its cleansing and astringent qualities enable Lemon to help reduce wrinkles, clear clogged pores and stimulate blood flow to the face.

If you are feeling a bit down or mentally fatigued use Lemon in a bath or burner to renew flagging energies. It helps to clear the brain, stimulate memory and enhance clarity.

Source:

Peel by expression

Properties:

- ➤ Antibacterial
- ➤ Antifungal
- ➤ Antiseptic
- ➤ Astringent
- ➤ Diuretic
- ➤ Detoxifying

<u>Uses</u>:

- ➤ Acne
- ➤ Arthritis
- ➤ Body Odour
- ➤ Cellulite
- ➤ Colds & Flu
- ➤ Cooling
- ➤ Detox
- ➤ Herpes
- ➤ High Blood Pressure
- ➤ Poor Circulation
- ➤ Prevents Infection
- ➤ Stimulates Digestive System
- ➤ Tonic for the Lymphatic System
- ➤ Wrinkles

<u>Caution</u>:

Avoid exposure to direct sun for 24 hours after application.

Marjoram (Origanum Marjorana)

Marjoram is an extremely versatile and useful essential oil. It has a strong warming quality so is very useful for all systems of the body which are sluggish – circulatory, lymphatic and digestive.

Use Marjoram in a massage blend for tight muscles or, if you have a tendency to cramping muscles, use it regularly to keep them at bay.

It is a helpful essential oil for high blood pressure so use it in a massage blend and massage the chest area, down the arms and the neck. If you suffer from carpel tunnel or repetitive strain syndrome try some Marjoram in a blend with other synergistic oils to relieve the symptoms and promote healing.

For digestive upsets it is handy for general indigestion, flatulence, colic or constipation.

Marjoram is an essential oil which is especially good for all those times when ladies need a helping hand to get through the menstrual pain or cramping – a gentle massage on the tummy area is very soothing.

If you have had a stressful day or one filled with anxiety and nervous tension, possibly resulting in a headache, try some Marjoram in a bath or as an inhalant. For times of grief or separation Marjoram is especially helpful to ease the heartache as it conveys a sense of comfort and support.

Source:

Dried leaves and flowers via distillation

Properties:

> Analgesic
> Antibacterial
> Antifungal
> Anti-viral
> Sedative

<u>Uses</u>:

- Asthma
- Aches
- Bruises
- Bronchitis
- Chilblains
- Colic
- Constipation
- Headaches
- High Blood Pressure
- Insomnia
- Menstrual Cramps
- Palpitations
- Sinusitis
- Spasms

Peppermint (Menthe Piperita)

Peppermint has been used for digestive complaints since it was first discovered by humans. Use it for all complaints of this system like indigestion, cramps, colic, flatulence, Irritable Bowel Syndrome (a massage would be effective here).

Peppermint's main active ingredient is menthol which is an effective decongestant. Menthol seems to be able to thin mucous so use Peppermint for all respiratory ailments such as sinusitis, bronchitis and asthma. Use an inhalant method for all upper respiratory conditions, and to relieve chest congestion use a compress or a massage.

Peppermint has a wonderful cooling effect on the skin and on our moods. It can be applied to all feverish or inflamed conditions of the skin, and if used in a facial spray (add a couple of drops to some water) it can help open up clogged pores.

You can use Peppermint to reduce bad breath, heal mouth ulcers or oral thrush by gargling a few drops dissolved in a glass of water.

In the house it is an effective pest deterrent against mice, fleas and ants.

As a mood enhancer it is fantastic to elevate our mood, clear the mind, eliminate negative thoughts, lessen mental fatigue and act as a general boost to our sometimes flagging energy levels.

Source:

Flowers via distillation

Properties:

> Anti-inflammatory
> Analgesic
> Digestive
> Expectorant
> Vasoconstrictor

<u>Uses</u>:

- Acne
- Bronchitis & Colds
- Bad Breath
- Catarrh
- Colic & Cramps
- Fatigue
- Flatulence
- Headaches
- Irritable Bowel Syndrome
- Insect Repellent
- Indigestion
- Nausea
- Period Pain
- Reduces Fever
- Rheumatism
- Sinusitis
- Toothache
- Varicose Veins

Rosemary (Rosmarinus Officinalis)

The Herb of Remembrance has been used for centuries in the sickroom as a fumigant and as a flea repellent because of its strong antiseptic qualities. But Rosemary has so many other vital uses in the modern world which warrants an inclusion in the 10 Best Essential Oils.

Rosemary is a stimulant, both physically and mentally, so it is excellent for refreshing the mind and body in a bath. Use it for stimulating the muscular system and easing tension in tight muscles in the back and legs, cramps, gout. It is useful in the circulatory system to stimulate blood and lymph flow which will help with varicose veins, fluid retention, osteoporosis, arthritis, and swelling.

This essential oil is excellent as a tonic, mainly for the liver and gall bladder and used in a massage blend can be beneficial for the digestive system.

Rosemary is wonderful in any topical or inhalant application for all the flu type symptoms. Use it for colds, flu, bronchitis, asthma, and sinusitis.

As Rosemary is a stimulant it is helpful for relieving fatigue, lethargy, exhaustion, and a tired mind. Place some drops in a burner or relax in a bath.

Source:

Flowering parts via distillation

Properties:

- ➢ Analgesic
- ➢ Antiseptic
- ➢ Astringent
- ➢ Decongestant
- ➢ Stimulant
- ➢ Tonic

<u>Uses</u>:

- Arthritis
- Asthma
- Chilblains
- Cramps
- Dandruff
- Flu
- Fumigant
- Infections
- Muscle Aches
- Lethargy
- Memory Aid
- Oily Skin
- Pest Repellent
- Poor Circulation
- Sciatica
- Sinusitis
- Sprains
- Tonic: Digestion, Liver, Gall Bladder
- Varicose Veins

Tea Tree (Melaleuca Alternifolia)

The antiseptic applications of this amazing essential oil are awesome. Who hasn't used Tea Tree for Athlete's Foot?

Its antifungal, anti-viral and antibacterial properties put it in a class of its own in my opinion.

Use it for all types of infections like acne, ringworm, sunburn, boils, cold sores, dandruff, pimples.

Use diluted in a sitz bath for all genito-urinary infections. This can include cystitis, vaginitis, candida.

Its anti-viral and antibacterial properties make it very useful for respiratory infections like the flu - make up a spray bottle with water and a few drops of Tea Tree and Lavender and spray the sickroom to help reduce fever and clear the air of bacteria.

Tea Tree is wonderful for bracing the spirit and improving self-confidence. It's an energy booster and general mood enhancer.

Source:

Leaves and twigs via distillation.

Properties:

- Antiseptic
- Antiviral
- Antifungal
- Antibiotic

Uses:

- Acne
- Athlete's Foot
- Boils
- Candida
- Cystitis
- Cold Sores
- Colds & Flu
- Dandruff
- Insect Bites and Repellent

- Nail Fungal Infections
- Mental Clarity
- Ringworm
- Sinusitis
- Sunburn
- Warts

Thyme (Thymus Vulgaris)

Thyme has been used for centuries as a healing and culinary plant.

However, it should be used in moderation in the healing arts as it is a strong stimulant to the thyroid and lymphatic system.

But because of its stimulant properties it is excellent for the immune system, bad breath, coughs/colds, mouth infections like gum disease (consult an Aromatherapist before using any internal dosages), an aid to recovery from illness.

Thyme has a hypertensive quality so it can help raise blood pressure.

It is known for its ability to remove toxins from the body, and you can use as a topical application for abscesses, burns and stings.

It is also good for warts, rheumatism, neuralgia, exhaustion and keeping the flying and biting nasties at bay!

Put some drops in a burner to soothe the mind, relax the soul, restore a sense of balance and help your body and spirit to heal after an illness or trauma.

Source:

Leaves and flowering parts via distillation.

Properties:

- ➢ Antioxidant
- ➢ Antibiotic
- ➢ Antiseptic
- ➢ Antiviral
- ➢ Anti-toxic
- ➢ Disinfectant

<u>Uses</u>:

- ➢ Acne
- ➢ Abscesses
- ➢ Bites & Stings
- ➢ Bronchitis
- ➢ Burns
- ➢ Coughs
- ➢ Cystitis
- ➢ Fatigue
- ➢ Flu
- ➢ Insect Repellent
- ➢ Immune System Stimulant
- ➢ Laryngitis
- ➢ Neuralgia
- ➢ Warts

<u>Cautions</u>:

- Do not over use as it can stimulate thyroid gland and lymphatic system
- Avoid if you have High Blood Pressure
- Do not use Red or Wild Thyme

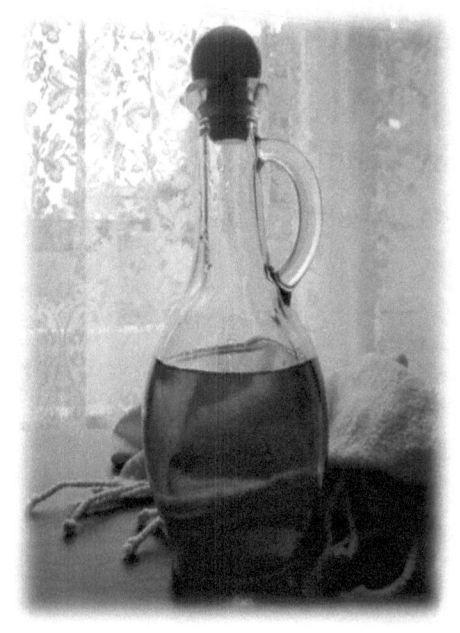

Chapter 3

The Carrier Oils

The majority of essential oils require a carrier before contact with the body.

Very few are applied directly as essential oils are highly concentrated and may adversely affect the skin.

If they are used in the bath then water is the carrier, if in a burner then the air is the carrier to our sense of smell, if in a massage then the massage oil is the carrier.

Dilution Ratios:

Drops	Millilitres of Carrier
1	1
<5	5
<10	10
<15	15
<20	20
<25	25
<30	30

The Main Carrier Oils:

➤ Almond, Sweet   (All Skin Types)

Contains vitamins A, B1, B2, B6 and E with a high protein content. It keeps reasonably well and because of the vitamin E is good for skin irritations.

➤ Avocado   (All Skin Types)

Contains vitamins A, B and D, lecithin and protein. It keeps very well but should be used in a dilution of 20% with 80% other oil. Especially good for wrinkles, skin irritations and dry skin.

➤ Evening Primrose   (All Skin Types)

Contains linoleic acid, vitamins and minerals. Keeps reasonably well but should be used in a dilution of 10% to 90% of other oil. Useful for heart disease, arthritis and premature ageing of the skin.

➤ Jojoba   (All Skin Types)

Contains myristic acid which is an anti-inflammatory. Keeps very well but should be used in a dilution of 10% to 90% of other oil. The chemical structure resembles sebum so it is excellent for treating inflamed skins, acne and dandruff.

➤ Sunflower   (All Skin Types)

Contains vitamins A, B, D and E. If it is obtained organically then it will keep quite well. Useful for bruises, leg ulcers and skin conditions. Suitable for all skin types.

➤ Wheatgerm   (All Skin Types)

Contains high levels of vitamin E. It keeps very well and is often used as a stabilising agent in other less well keeping oils at a ratio of 10% wheatgerm to the other oil. For massage and essential oil blend it should be used in a dilution of 20% with 80% other oil. Especially good for eczema and prematurely ageing skin.

Chapter 4

The Ten Best Essential Oils

Properties Chart

Name	Antibiotic	Antiseptic	Anti-Viral	Anti-Fungal	Anti-Inflammatory
Chamomile	✓	✓			
Eucalyptus	✓	✓	✓	✓	
Geranium		✓			✓
Lavender	✓	✓	✓	✓	✓
Lemon	✓	✓		✓	
Marjoram		✓			
Peppermint		✓			✓
Rosemary		✓			
Tea Tree	✓	✓	✓	✓	
Thyme	✓	✓	✓	✓	

Essential Oils can help

heal our ailments,

soothe our nerves,

uplift our moods,

ease sore muscles,

clear up acne,

relieve stress,

enhance our libido,

relax our bodies in massage,

induce sleep,

cleanse the air we breathe,

disinfect our pets' bedding,

clean our homes and

keep our gardens pest free

all without chemicals…

Notes